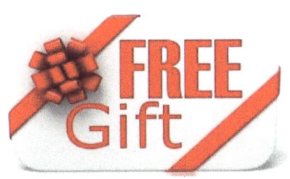

Want Priority Access to FREE eBooks Additional Materials for this Book?

As we release NEW eBooks, we offer them for FREE for a limited time. You will be the FIRST one to know when they are FREE. Join 1000's of insiders who are getting access to FREE Kindle book promotions weekly.

Click HERE for FREE additional material and FREE eBooks-
www.rictamilypublishing.com

Table of Contents

Introduction

I want to thank you and congratulate you for downloading the book, *"Slimming Secretes: Health, Fitness, and Diet Secrets for the New You"*.

Losing weight is not an easy task that a lot of people have to deal with. Maintaining a healthy weight is another burden that people carry. False advertisements and ineffective diet plans are often misleading and tricky. It's frustrating to waste time, effort, and money for fake diet programs.

There came a time where fitness and physical activity became a popular method to lose weight instead of dieting. However, it was another moneymaking scheme to make people enroll in a fitness class and pay for a gym membership. This method needs extreme training and demands time and patience for effective results.

A single method is not sufficient to induce weight loss or maintain a healthy weight. Why is that so? – Because weight problems like obesity are multifactorial in origin. There are different factors that cause a person to gain weight. Therefore, a single weight loss method is not the answer that you are looking for.

The weight loss secrets in this book are a compilation of scientific evidences that nutritionists and health experts use. My approach is a holistic weight loss program for a total and long lasting fitness. Losing weight is not just about dieting and exercising, but rather it's a skill that uses varied methods to solve the multifactorial cause of weight gain.

In this book, you will learn about the principles of healthy dieting, the appropriate workout for your body type, and how to avoid the common weight loss pitfalls that people encounter. The book also offers solutions for the body's metabolism, hormone regulation, and rest cycle. These are additional benefits that the book provides, since these are not usually tackled in other slimming programs.

Included is an easy step-by-step guide on how to lose 15 kilos or more in just eight weeks. This is attainable by using a holistic approach for a total body makeover. These weight loss secrets are not new but are based on a compilation of scientific evidences. My fun and stress-free approach to weight loss hopefully would guide you into a healthier and slimmer body that you long for. Again, thank you for downloading and I wish you best of luck with this weight loss secret.

Chapter 1
The Secret behind Different Diet Plans

People often have a hard time choosing a diet regimen to follow since there are lots of diet regimens available in the market. What's most important is to follow a diet regimen that will fit your lifestyle and personality so that it would work. In this chapter you will learn about the different principles used by diet plans. You will get surprised that most of them follow the same concept.

Step One: *Set a target weight, the higher – the better!*

Before starting on anything, take note of your body weight and your waist circumference as well. Compute for your current body mass index (BMI) and set a body weight that you want to achieve. Don't be shy to aim for a higher weight loss because the higher your goal is, the better result you will get. Challenge yourself and don't settle for less, remember that motivation and hard work is the key to success.

Now let's plan to reach your target weight in eight weeks. For example, a woman who is 5'4" tall and weighs 170 pounds have a target weight of 140 pounds after eight weeks. Distribute the 30 pound weight loss over the eight week program. This principle of rapid weight loss is used by diet programs because of its effectiveness and long term benefit. Don't let the numbers intimidate you, you'll get more motivated once you see rapid and big results.

Step Two: *Saturated versus unsaturated fat, know the difference.*

Removing unhealthy fat is another principle used by all diet plans. Saturated fats are unhealthy which directly increase blood cholesterol and LDL levels. Polyunsaturated and monounsaturated fats are healthy fat recommended by health professionals because they sweep off bad cholesterol and lipids.

Removing unhealthy fat and promoting the good fat are seen in Weight Watchers Diet, Mayo Clinic Diet, South Beach Diet, and Paleo Diet. You can also try this principle by choosing foods rich in healthy fats like corn oil, olive oil, soybean, safflower, canola oil, and fish. Nutritious fish to remember are HAMMS: **H**erring, **A**nchovies, **M**ackerel, **S**almon, and **S**ardines. You can also snack on nuts and avocados; they're rich in good fat too.

Step Three: *Choose complex carbohydrates over simple sugar.*

Complex carbohydrates provide more nutritional value than simple carbohydrates. If you try to notice most of the diet plans contain complex carbohydrates because they also contain fiber for improved digestion. Simple carbohydrates on the other hand, are rapidly digested, which can make you feel hungry even after intake.

Try this principle by choosing foods rich in complex carbohydrates like green vegetables, whole grains, beans, and peas. These are rich in vitamins, minerals, fiber, and complex carbohydrates. You have a wide variety to choose from, which can satisfy your appetite. Avoid diet sodas since they contain sugar substitute that are not good for your health.

Step Four: *What fits your personality and lifestyle is best.*

After knowing which food to choose, we now put these principles into action. Diet programs have been claiming their superiority over the others when it comes to weight loss. A Canadian compilation of over 59 credible journals says that diet programs bring the same result. The weight loss difference between diet programs was minimal and not significant. The bottom line is to go on a diet and choose a program that best fit your lifestyle. You can eat the food that you like provided that it's healthy.

Step Five: *The secret formula on how to reach your goal*

In order to lose 1-1.5 kilos per week, you need to reduce 1,000 calories from your daily intake. If your goal is to lose 0.5 kilo per week, you'll need to reduce 500 calories from your daily intake. Decreasing daily calorie intake is one thing diet programs have in common because fewer intake will ultimately lead to weight loss. These are true if you choose to go on a diet without exercise. The formula is suitable for people who don't have enough time to enroll in an exercise program.

In this chapter we have discussed the basic principles for dieting and maintaining a healthy weight. The right food choices were also discussed to prevent you from committing common weight loss mistakes. The planning phase is done; now let's move on how you can apply these principles to reach your goal. The next chapter will help you understand proper dieting without having rebound effects.

Chapter 2
Food Science: Slimming without Rebound Effects

The time of food intake is likewise important in dieting. It has a direct effect of the body's hormonal regulation and metabolism. In this chapter you will learn about how meal frequency and time affects body metabolism and hormonal regulation.

You might wonder why your diet isn't working; a probable answer is that you could be doing something wrong. Trying to be slim and lose weight does not only involve the type and amount of food that you take. Here are three things to keep in mind when you want to be slimmer:

Don't skip meals – Skipping meals, especially breakfast would make you overeat throughout the day. Eating a healthy breakfast keeps your metabolism going. It even prolongs satiety and reduces food cravings. The calories you ate for breakfast will be used through the day and will not be stored as fat. Skipping meals is a big no-no since it causes overeating and rebound weight gain.

Time of meals – Eating five small meals in a day is better than three bulky meals. Small amounts for more frequency keep your metabolism going. This also prevents the release of "ghrelin", the hunger hormone. As a result, eating five small meals in a day can decrease your appetite. When you eat, it is also important to take your time and enjoy your meal. Chew your food thoroughly, there's no need to rush when eating. Eating slowly promotes the feeling of being full and satisfied.

Enjoy dieting, but stay focused – People who enjoy dieting and do it at their own pace experience better results. Frustration and stress that accompany dieting leads to non-compliance or emotional-eating. Stay focused, eat healthy, and have fun as you work your way to the new you.

These three methods, improve your eating behavior as you learn about how the body reacts with meals. Skipping of meals, especially breakfast is a big no-no. The timing and frequency of meals actually keep the metabolism going and trains the body to control appetite. With these, you lose weight without worrying about gaining the kilos back. In the next chapter, we will discuss on other ways to prolong your satiety and reduce appetite.

Chapter 3
The Power of Proteins

Protein is a best friend of body builders and dieters as well. Taking enough amount of protein would even help you maintain a lean body figure. Women most commonly ignore protein in their diet and choose carbohydrates and vegetables instead. This chapter will help you understand the benefits of eating protein.

Benefits of Eating Protein

1. Helps in the recovery of muscles after exercise

Almost all bodily structures are made of protein and the body naturally uses protein to build and repair tissues. If your muscles are sore after exercise or you have a wound, protein will help speed up your recovery. This macronutrient also helps maintain the integrity of bones, skin, hair, and all types of muscles.

2. Builds lean muscles

Protein rich foods with a high biological value promote a lean body structure. This is true for people who want to lose body fat and be fit. For body builders, they do need to take higher amounts of protein. Building lean muscles are important while dieting. When people go on a diet, the body breaks down protein as a response to the restricted caloric intake. Incorporating quality protein in the diet prevents this response. Dieting with protein also reduces common down side of weight loss which is having loose skin on the belly, sides, and arms.

3. Helps in maintaining a healthy weight

Protein is actively used by the body, in excess it does not accumulate in fats. Instead, it is used by the body to synthesize hormones, enzymes, essential amino acids. Protein is a basic nutrient used by most diet programs because of its support in maintaining a healthy body weight. It boosts metabolism by sparing the muscles and allows the body to use fat stores instead.

4. Curbs hunger

Proteins keep your body lean and strong. The stomach takes a long time to digest protein that is why it can prolong satiety and reduce food cravings. You can feel a decrease in appetite within 2-4 days of eating quality protein. Combining protein with fiber can naturally and effectively solve food cravings similar to slimming pills.

Amount of Protein Consumption

The recommended daily allowance for protein is 0.8gm per kilo of body weight in order to maintain a healthy weight. A 70 kg man would need 56gm daily protein. Body builders need to consult nutritionists or experts on how much protein to add to their diet.

IMPORTANT: Eating excess protein and going over the recommended daily allowance is not advantageous. It damages the kidneys and the excess protein undergoes deamination for fat synthesis.

Protein with High Biologic Value

Quality protein means that it has a lot of biological value and amino acids. Proteins from meat, fish, poultry, and milk have high biologic value compared to protein derived from plants. They offer complete amino acids essential for the body. Listed below are protein rich foods you can use as a guide.

Foods with Quality Protein

- Fish: Yellow Fin Tuna, Halibut, Salmon, Tilapia
- Poultry: Chicken Breast, Turkey Breast

- Meat: Pork Chops, Lean Beef and Veal, Steak (Top of Bottom Round)
- Vegetables: Beans, Tofu, Legumes
- Canned foods: Anchovies, Sardines
- Snacks: Nuts, Seeds
- Dairy: Milk, Cheese, Eggs, Yogurt, Soy Milk and Soy products

Protein is a powerful nutrient that can help the body lose weight, build lean muscles, and maintain a healthy weight. It is also helpful for people who have a hard time controlling their food cravings. Eating foods with quality protein are recommended. The chapter further discussed other benefits of eating protein and its effect on the body. Other slimming tips are discussed in the next chapter, emphasizing on how to speed up the body's metabolism and lose more weight.

Chapter 4
How to Boost Metabolism and Lose More Weight

Faster metabolism helps the body lose more weight; it even speeds up the weight reduction process. There are several ways of speeding up the body's metabolism. Exercise is not the only way that can boost metabolism. As a matter of fact, there is a concept known as diet-induced thermogenesis (metabolism). In this chapter you will learn about how to boost your metabolism using diet-induced thermogenesis.

Caffeine

Coffee: 16% increase in metabolism

The effect of coffee on basal metabolic rate is proven through different researches. According to a recent study conducted, people who drank caffeinated coffee resulted to increase in their metabolic rate over those who drank decaf. Coffee offers a maximum of 16 percent increase in the body's metabolic rate.

Doctors and nutrition experts say that coffee stimulates the sympathetic nervous system. As a result, the heart rate and respiratory rate increase and burns more calories. However, be conscious of your coffee intake. Don't splurge on frappe and other drinks with added sugar and whip cream.

Red Chili Pepper & Ginger

Red Chili Pepper: 8% increase in metabolism

Ginger: 20% increase in metabolism

Red chili pepper and ginger are spices that can speed up metabolism. According to the *New York Times*, red chili pepper contains capsaicin; this chemical component of chili generates heat in the body. It even burn more calories right after eating a spicy meal. Enjoying a spicy meal increases metabolism by eight percent.

Another research conducted in Canada also says that appetizers with hot sauce results to 200 calorie consumption during the day. This was due to the effect of capsaicin in increasing and prolonging satiety. Do take caution when eating spicy foods, especially on an empty stomach, since it can worsen heartburn and ulcer symptoms.

Green Tea

3 cups Green tea: 10% increase in metabolism

Green tea is loaded with antioxidants that reduce free radicals in the body. It also contains catechin which is the primarily responsible in boosting metabolism. Nutritionists and researchers explain the catechin works by promoting fat oxidation and enhancing thermogenesis. It helps promote and maintain weight loss by improving digestion.

Cinnamon

¼ - 1 tsp. Cinnamon: 20% increase in metabolism

Cinnamon is not just a regular spice, it can also help you lose more weight and increase your metabolism. It works by directly affecting the regulation of insulin in your body. Insulin is the hormone which influences the metabolism of fat and carbohydrates. During the process, it also increases the body's metabolic rate and energy expenditure.

Berries

You can snack on raspberries and strawberries. These are known to contain antioxidants and chemicals that speed up the body's metabolic rate. These red berries contain anthocyanins; these are biochemical that eliminates fat cells in the body. In addition, they work by affecting glucose metabolism.

The *Journal of Nutrition and Metabolism* published in 2014 more options for you to choose from, they are: lingonberries, bilberries, and blackcurrants. These berries contain quercetin glycosides which significantly reduces body fat. Quercetin glycosides are also known for preventing or blocking the metabolic effects of a high-fat diet.

In conclusion, the chapter discussed about five types of food that naturally burn fat and increase the body's metabolic rate. Don't get overwhelmed with the facts and try them all at the same time. You can try red chili pepper for Monday and ginger for Tuesday. Add variation and have fun as you naturally increase your metabolism. Eat snacks loaded with fiber, protein, or good fat can also rev up your metabolism. The chapter focused on increasing your metabolism as a supplement for weight loss. The next chapter will also discuss about other weight loss tips you can use to maximize your diet program.

Chapter 5
Weight Loss Myths Revealed

The way to have a slimmer body is hard and most people get attracted to promises of easy weight loss. Focus, motivation, and self-discipline are the core values that people need to have a healthy body. In the previous chapters, we discussed about the basic principles on how to lose weight. In this chapter you will discover about different weight loss myths and how you should handle them.

Weight Loss Myths

1. Cutting out snacks will help you lose weight.

Snacking is okay, if you eat healthy snacks and would consume only what you need. Avoid snacks that are high in saturated fat and sugar. Eating fruits and nuts would help your metabolism going.

2. Slimming pills are effective for long term weight loss.

Slimming pills alone are either act as diuretics or laxatives. They do not really help you control your eating behavior; instead it gives people the freedom of consuming a lot of calories thinking that it won't add up to their weight.

3. Foods with "reduced-fat" or "less-fat" labels are healthy.

These labels could be misleading and are not healthy options. The US Food and Drug Administration says that these items are added with salt, flour, sugar, or starch to improve the flavor and texture after the fat is removed. As a result, these foods actually contain more calories than the full-fat version

4. Others can eat whatever they want and still lose weight.

Eating alone is just a part of losing weight. People can eat whatever they want to provide that they burn more calories than their food intake in order to lose weight.

5. Lifting weights will only produce a bigger body built.

The right combination of exercise will help people lose weight faster. As a matter of fact, the combination of aerobics and weight lifting exercises will speed up the weight loss process because of the added energy expenditure.

6. Physical activity only works if I do it for a longer duration.

If you try to look at books and other reference, physical activity is recommended on a weekly basis. Experts would rather recommend aerobic exercise or a high intensity workout for more than 10 minutes.

7. Eating meat will not help me lose weight.

Lean meat will help you form a leaner body structure. Meat also contains a lot of nutrients like protein, iron, and zinc. Lean meat takes a longer time to be digested and helps control a person's appetite.

8. Dairy products are fattening.

Low-fat cheese, milk, and yogurt are nutritious and contain fewer calories than whole milk dairy products. These will not make you fatter, but they will help you build a strong and slim body.

9. Going vegetarian will help lose more weight.

Three different kinds of vegetarian diet that people follow. For people starting on a vegetarian diet, they tend to crave for food with more calories and less nutrients. Most people, who were not originally vegetarians, go back to their usual diet and regain their weight.

10. One weight loss regimen is good enough.

Overweight and obesity are caused by different factors. Using one weight loss regimen is not adequate to address the varied factors that affect weight.

In this chapter, we discussed the different weight loss myths that most people actually do. It is important to use scientific evidences when losing weight instead of just applying misleading advertisements and rumors. These ten myths are backed up with research and scientific evidences. In the next chapter, we will discuss about physical activities that will help you lose more weight.

Chapter 6
Understanding Different Levels of Activity – How to Use Them with Dieting

While dieting, you restrict your body with the calories and energy intake. Inactivity or sedentary lifestyle combined with dieting will only slow down your metabolism. It is a natural response of the body to compensate with the decreased caloric intake. On the other hand, the severe physical activity might destroy your diet and could even lead to overeating. In this chapter, you will learn about the different levels of activity and how to use them while you are on a diet.

Moderate Intensity Exercises at First

As you start a diet program, your body also adjusts to the change in your daily intake. Your metabolism could slow down as a result of dieting. In the initial phase of the weight loss program, you need to start with moderate activity and gradually introduce vigorous activity. Here are some examples of moderate intensity exercises:

- Brisk walking
- Heavy cleaning or mowing the lawn
- Light bicycling
- Badminton
- Tennis (doubles)
- Table tennis
- Dancing

It is best to start with moderate intensity activities because these are sufficient enough to make the body burn more calories. These types of activities burn 3 to 6 times more energy per minute compared to your regular activities.

Vigorous Intensity Exercise for Maintenance

As your body adapts with the type of physical activity, you can gradually increase the level of difficulty to challenge yourself even more. This level of physical activity is recommended when you're in the middle phase of weight loss program. You should consider vigorous exercises since these types of activities burn over 7 to 10 times more energy per minute.

Here are some examples of moderate intensity exercises:

- Jogging/running
- Cycling uphill
- Hiking, rock climbing
- Tennis (singles)
- Basketball or soccer (game)
- Swimming

Experts say that ten minutes of high intensity training is enough for the day. This is recommended, especially for people who are on a diet. Vigorous physical activity leads to overeating, stress, and frustration. In addition, don't do extreme exercises for 2 to 3 consecutive days. Give time for your body to heal and rest.

How to determine moderate from vigorous intensity exercises?

People have different lifestyles and activities of daily living. Thus, a moderate exercise for teenagers may not be considered as moderate in intensity for an adult. Breathing is one measure to determine if you're burning enough calories.

Generally, in moderate intensity exercises you can still talk and catch your breath. Some people can sing with their workout playlist. In contrast, you can't sing during the activity if you're doing vigorous intensity exercises. You can only say a few words at this level of activity. Difficulty of breathing and light headedness is symptoms indicating that you need to reduce the level of physical activity.

To wrap it up, moderate level of physical activities is best during the initial phase of the weight loss program. You can gradually increase the difficulty depending on how fast your body adapts and recover. Pay attention to your breathing so you can determine if you need to level up or reduce the physical activity. Make sure to rehydrate and rest after your workout. In the next chapter, we will further discuss on workout programs for different body types.

Chapter 7
Physical Activity for your Body Type

Many people who try popular workouts should understand that certain types of exercises are more effective depending on their body type. In this chapter you will learn about the workout that best fit your body type. You will also learn about how to get slim body versus a sexy body.

Pear Shaped Body

People with a pear shaped body have excess body fat distributed over the lower half of their body. The common areas of concern are the hips, butt, and thighs. To solve excessive fat distribution in the lower body, you need to tone the gluts and the thighs.

Exercises like brisk walking, jogging, or dancing will help you lose more weight and reduce body fat stored in your hips and thighs. Add it with strength training to burn more fats and develop lean muscles at the same time. You can also start toning the butt and thigh areas after losing some weight. Toning will help tighten the skin around these areas and prevent loose skin.

People with a pear shaped body are lucky because it is easier to lose weight for their body type. You also need to strengthen your core, arms, and shoulders to balance your figure. Although it sounds ironic, but paying attention to the areas above the waist will camouflage a pear shaped body type.

Apple Shaped Body

People with an apple shaped body have more fat distributed over waist and are rounder in the middle. The common areas of concern include the belly and waistline. Abdominal exercises and high intensity exercises would help solve people with a wide waistline and a muffin top.

Cardio exercises are best at removing abdominal fat, according to a study conducted at Duke University. However, jogging and cycling are not recommended for people with an apple shaped body type. Jogging will exhaust the muscles in the legs and thighs because of a heavier upper body. As a result, they force the muscles in the legs to get bigger in order to carry the weight as they jog.

Cycling focuses on different muscle groups and it does not solve the fatty areas in an apple shaped body. In order to get a slim and beautiful body, you need to work on the abdominal muscles and the oblique muscles. Belly dancing, jump rope, bicycle crunch, and the hula hoop are good activities that focus on the waist and hip area.

Straight Body Frame

Some people do have a straight body frame and long for more curves or more bulk. People with a straight frame need to focus on toning or building more muscles depending on their goal. Body sculpting could be achieved with resistance exercises using resistance bands or weights.

Strength and resistance training are recommended for men who want to build more muscle. The guide in body sculpting is to focus on the area where you need more shape. Body sculpting and muscle building would often take weeks to bring noticeable results. Be patient, the muscles do take time to get in shape.

Hourglass Body Frame

People with an hourglass body frame have fat distributed both on the upper and lower areas of the body. Although they have a small appearing waist, they do have areas of concern like the upper arms, belly pooch, and thighs.

Aerobic exercises like dancing and swimming could help solve fat distributed throughout the body. Other forms of exercise that work for both upper and lower areas could also help you gain a fit and toned hourglass body.

Knowing your body type and areas of concern are essential in choosing the kind of exercise to incorporate into your weight loss program. For example, jogging is good for those who have a pear shaped body, but is not advisable for people with an apple shaped body. We discussed about the different body types and the exercises that can solve the common areas of concern. In the next chapter, we will discuss about the effects of rest and relaxation and how these help in the slimming process.

Chapter 8
Rest and Relaxation – How it Helps in the Slimming Process

In the previous chapters we have discussed about the several ways and methods on how to get a beautiful body that you long for. The facts and details discussed could get overwhelming and stressing. Losing weight is not just about self-discipline and exercising, you also need to rest and let your body relax as you get closer to your goal. In this chapter, you will learn about the benefits of relaxation techniques and how it helps your body in the slimming process.

Sauna

Many studies do support the positive effect of the sauna when it comes to weight loss. These scientific evidences make it more fun to use the sauna for both slimming and relaxation. The persistent heat generated by sauna directly increases the body's core temperature. Thus, the increased body temperature also results in a transient increase in the body's metabolism.

The increase in heart rate and perspiration are the most evident signs that sauna boosts the body's metabolism. Using the sauna has a similar effect to mild exercise. In fact, one sauna session can burn 350 – 500 calories! A sauna bath helps the body relax, detoxify, relieve stress, and lose weight all at the same time. Experts recommend using the sauna after a workout for more effective results.

Meditation

Meditation is another popular relaxation technique that is beneficial for mental, physical, and emotional health. It creates a strong connection between body and mind.

Aside from its stress relieving effect, meditation also helps in weight management, brain functioning, and disease prevention.

With sufficient practice, meditation and breathing techniques help in weight management by reducing the urge to eat. It helps the mind focus and concentrate on the weight loss program. Meditate, breathe, and count to ten whenever you have food cravings. Ask yourself if you're really hungry or is it just emotional eating.

Eating behaviors are not addressed by most weight loss programs. This is the reason why people find it hard to maintain weight loss. As you develop the correct mantra and breathing technique, you also build a mindful eating where you consider eating as a healthy choice and not as a habit. Meditate for 30 minutes in a day and feel the greatest connection between your body and mind.

Sleep

Sleep for six to eight hours and reward yourself for all the hard work you've accomplished during the day. Getting enough sleep recharges your body and it also reduces the production of hormones responsible for overeating.

Sleep deprivation causes weight gain because lack of sleep affects hormone regulation and metabolic processes in the body. That is why sleep and rest is important to keep the metabolic processes balanced. Sleep was even featured in *the Dr. Oz show,* as a way of controlling hormone levels and reducing weight.

Studies also show that people who slept for six to eight hours had the lower body mass index than those who were deprived of sleep. So rest and sleep, it's good for your mind, health, and weight.

Rest and relaxation techniques are also beneficial for weight loss and eliminating bad eating habits. Other relaxation techniques like yoga, massage, and tai chi are also beneficial for overall wellness. The connection between the mind and body are often neglected in weight loss programs. However, rest and relaxation are equally important for people who want to lose weight. We have discussed about the benefits of relaxation when it comes to losing weight. In the next chapter, we will discuss on how to incorporate various weight loss methods into your personal slimming plan.

Chapter 9
Advantage of Using Various Slimming Methods

We have discussed different slimming methods; now let us use that knowledge into a weight loss program that best fit your lifestyle, personality, and body type. No single slimming method is effective; keep in mind that combining different techniques are proven to be more effective. In this chapter you will learn about how to use variety in your weight loss program and why it is important in the slimming process.

Variety in Your Personal Weight Loss Program

Dieting alone or exercising alone could give partially effective results. But the combination of diet, exercise, and relaxation techniques will definitely cut more weight and body fat. Keep in mind that weight is multifactorial and losing weight is a skill where you focus on the different aspects of weight and health.

The mind and body are good at adapting to sudden changes including weight loss. Severe caloric restriction will work initially, but will no longer be effective once the body have adjusted with your self-imposed calorie restriction.

The same is also true for exercise or physical activity. Doing the same routine will make you sweat less as you get accustomed to performing the same activity over and over again. Varying the intensity, duration, and frequency of your workout plan will help you burn more calories and lose more weight.

Mindful Eating

As discussed in the first chapter, no diet program is significantly more effective than the others. Different researches were compiled to show that diet programs are equally effective. Therefore, it is important to go on a plan that you will follow. Don't waste your time following a regimen that you're not happy with.

Go with what suits you best, it will lead to more compliance and successful results. What's important is that you know the principles behind diet programs that we've discussed. Here are more tips as you go through the slimming process:

- Using a food diary (daily or weekly) to guide you in making necessary adjustments.
- Count to ten, do breathing exercises, or drink water every time you have the urge to eat.
- Eat when you're hungry and not when you're depressed or stressed out.
- Enjoy your food every meal and avoid multitasking. Avoid eating while watching TV or surfing the net.

Listen to your body

Enter an exercise regimen that you enjoy and makes you happy. Physical activity could be done in different forms and should not be limited to gym memberships. Your exercise routine and physical activity should be fun and not too tiring. Here are some reminders before you do slimming exercises:

- If your body is tired, take a rest and do a different activity.
- Don't use workout as an excuse to overeat.
- Don't use dieting as an excuse for inactivity.
- Incorporate different slimming methods to attain balance in your weight loss regimen.

Losing weight is not an easy task to do, however, it should not be stressful and tiring. Have fun as you gain more control over your eating habits. Weight is multifactorial and it is okay to use different slimming methods. We have discussed about the different aspects of weight and health. Get ready to welcome the new you, as we discuss in the next chapter final tips to keep in mind for a holistic and successful weight loss.

Chapter 10
Welcome the New You

Losing weight is not only about dieting or exercising. There are things that could either help or destroy your weight loss program. You will realize that you do have weight loss buddies and struggles as you work towards the goal. In this chapter you will know your weight loss buddies as you welcome your new body.

The final ingredients that you need:

1. Know your weight loss buddies

Every person has different struggles and challenges when it comes to weight loss. Self-discipline, motivation, and optimism are more powerful than any slimming pill or diet cookbook. You do know your own limitations, strengths, and motivating influences. And you do have all the control over your mind and body.

2. Conquer your limitations

Don't be afraid to go to the gym or enroll in a workout class just because of what others might think. Others will even be proud of you, especially your friends and family when they see all your hard work. Don't let fear and insecurities block your way. Health and fitness are for everybody and certainly, you too can have a fit and beautiful body.

3. Stay focused and motivated

Having a good plan and a food diary would help monitor your calorie intake and energy expenditure. Listing your daily achievements like your exercise during the day and less food cravings will also help you stay motivated. The people who monitor their progress do better and attain successful results. Monitoring is not just about weighing yourself daily, but you also need to reflect on your effort and compare it with the result.

4. Reward yourself

Say goodbye to the habit of rewarding yourself through food. Instead, reward yourself for your weight loss accomplishments like watching a movie or going to a spa. Feeling good about your body and is very empowering. You can also treat yourself after achieving a minor goal like getting a new dress after losing a few inches around your waist. You did a great job, so you might as well show off the result of your hard work.

Keep in mind that the will and motivating factor to have a new body comes from within. Mind what you eat, stay active, and get enough sleep. Do measures to keep your metabolism going. Chart your progress and challenge yourself to keep going as you get closer to your goal. Use appropriate physical activity for your body type.

Dieting and exercising could be fun, especially if it suits your lifestyle and personality. Maintain balance as much as possible and take care of your health. Take a rest and relax if you need to, they are good for your health and weight.

The real secret of health and fitness comes from within. Know your limitations and accept them. Use your strengths and the things that you've learned in this book. Remember, that the most powerful slimming weapon is YOU.

Conclusion

The mind and body have a strong connection that people can use in order to maintain a healthy weight. Don't focus on dieting alone or exercising alone. Set your goals and challenge yourself. Eat right, get enough sleep, and perform physical activity appropriate for your body type. There are lots of ways on how effectively to lose weight. Widen your perspective using these weight loss secrets and you will certainly enjoy the different benefits.

Thank you again for downloading this book!

I hope this book was able to help you lose body fat and maintain a healthy weight.

Share these weight loss secrets to your loved ones and help them feel the difference!

Review Link

If you enjoyed this book, we would really appreciate it if you could leave us a positive REVIEW?

P.S. **You can CLICK HERE to go directly to the book page** and leave your review and/or purchase our other books above. Alternatively, you can copy and paste this address into your browser --- http://amzn.to/1wCj3OE

Preview of, "10 Things You Need to Know about Ebola" Facts about the Virus, Symptoms, Quarantine and Prevention

The Ebola virus was first isolated and identified to 1976 in the Democratic Republic of Congo. This virus has been found to have an average mortality rate of 88 percent in humans, one of the highest recorded. Since its initial discovery, cases of Ebola fever have been identified and quarantined across central Africa.

The virus is spread by contact of bodily fluids and blood from others who are infected. Currently there are no documented cases of the virus spreading through the air. When this virus is contracted, individuals will start to show symptoms such as muscle pain, fever, headache or sore throat 2 days to 3 weeks later. This will be followed by rash, vomiting, diarrhea, decrease in kidney and liver function as well as internal and external bleeding. Prevention of these diseases focuses on decreasing the spread of the virus from animals to humans as there is not currently a treatment for this disease.

Ebola Virus Disease History

2014 Ebola Outbreak in West Africa

According to the most recent CDC outbreak information the countries of Nigeria, Guinea, Liberia and Sierra Leone are seeing one of the largest outbreaks of Ebola in world history. The Emergency Operations center is providing assistance and public health experts are working to expand resources to help control the outbreak. As of 20th August, more than 1400 people have died.

2012 Ebola Outbreak in Uganda (December)

In December 2012, 7 cases of Ebola were confirmed in the Luwero District of Uganda which caused 4 deaths. The Ministry of Health diagnosed and managed the outbreak with assistance from the Viral Special Pathogens Branch. The total numbers from this outbreak are expected to change.

2012 Ebola Outbreak in the Democratic Republic of Congo (November)

The DRC Ministry of Health declared an outbreak of Ebola in the Province Orientale on November 26, 2012. This outbreak included 77 cases confirmed by the CDC lab in Uganda which included 36 confirmed cases, 17 probable cases, 36 deaths and 24 suspected cases. The Public Health Agency of Canada provided additional diagnostic support for this outbreak.

2012 Ebola Outbreak in Uganda (July)

In July 2012, an outbreak of Ebola Hemorrhagic Fever in Kibaale Uganda was confirmed by the Uganda Ministry of Health. This included 24 probable human cases which are being researched at the Uganda Virus research Institute as well as the U.S. Centers for Disease Control and Prevention via blood sample. This outbreak has 11 confirmed patients with 4 deaths.

2011 Ebola Case in Uganda (May)

In May 2011 an outbreak of Ebola hemorrhagic fever was confirmed in the Luwero district of Uganda by the Ugandan Ministry of Health. Tests for the virus on blood samples confirmed the outbreak at the Uganda Viral Research Institute. To date, no additional cases have been reported.

2008 Ebola-Reston Virus Was Detected in Pigs in the Philippines

In October 2008 samples of tissue from pigs from the Philippines was tested by the Foreign Animal Disease Diagnostic Laboratory. These samples were taken from Manila where swine pathogens of the Ebola virus were identified using molecular analysis. This was the first time the Reston version of the virus was identified in pigs. An ongoing search is commencing to ensure that this virus was not spread to humans.

2007 Ebola Outbreak in the Democratic Republic of Congo

In August 2007 the Kasai Occidental Province was struck with a disease of unknown origins. Samples from the victims were sent to the CDC Special Pathogens Branch as well as the Centre International de Recherches Medicales de Franceville. Real time testing confirmed these cased to be from the Ebola virus, though the presence of other pathogens implies that additional diseases may have been present. This outbreak had a confirmed 249 cases resulting in 183 deaths.

2004 Ebola Outbreak in South Sudan

The World Health Organization confirmed 20 cases of Ebola hemorrhagic fever in Yambio County of south Sudan in 2004. This outbreak included 5 deaths which were studied by the Kenya Medical Research Institute and the Centers for Disease control. It was also confirmed that the strain which caused the outbreak was one previously known to cause human disease.

2003 Ebola Cases in the Democratic Republic of Congo

In 2003 several cases of Ebola hemorrhagic fever syndrome were confirmed by the World Health Organization Communicable Disease Surveillance and Response team in the Republic of the Congo.

2002 Ebola Outbreak in Gabon and Republic of the Congo

In May 2002, an outbreak of Ebola hemorrhagic fever was confirmed in the Ogooue Ivindo province by the Gabonese Ministry of Health and the World Health Organization. A response team was sent to this area and neighboring villages in the Republic of the Congo.

2001 Ebola Outbreak in Uganda

An outbreak of Ebola hemorrhagic fever which occurred over 42 days occurred in Uganda. It was officially declared over on February 27, 2001 after a period of time considered twice the maximum incubation period when no new cases were reported. Between October 2000-February 2001 the World Health Organization partnered with the CDC to help control the outbreak.

If you like this preview, then *click here for the full story of this eBook!*

Or go to: *http://www.amazon.com/dp/B00PQS7WDE/*

Check Out My Other Books

Anti-Cancer Diet: The Ultimate Guide in Fighting Cancer, Lowering Cancer Risks and Achieving Optimum Health

Liver Cleanse and Detox Diet: The Ultimate Guide in Cleansing the Body, Eliminating Toxins and Losing Weight!

Pilates for Beginners: The Essential Guide to Total Body Fitness, Strong Muscles and Lean Body

Anger, Stress and Fear: Your Personal Guide in Controlling Anger, Managing Stress and Overcoming Fear

Israel vs. the World: The Apple of God's Eye in the End times

Gilgamesh: King in Quest of Immortality – An Extra Biblical Proof for the Genesis Flood

Herbal Soap Making: How to Make Homemade Herbal Soaps that Clean and Nurture the Body!

Teeth Healing through Oil Pulling: The Complete Guide in Natural Oral Care through the Benefits of Oil Pulling

The Ad: A Mail-Order Bride Romance Series

Ultimate Guide to Financial Freedom: Achieve Wealth, Attain Success and Manage your Debt Like the Rich!

Dedication

To our three blessings that have made RicTamily complete and continue to grow together in His loving embrace.

Disclaimer

The information in this book is in no way intended as medical advice. This book is not meant to be used, nor should it be used, to diagnose or treat any medical condition. The author disclaims responsibility for any adverse health effects that come in combination with the use of methods and suggestions presented in the book. The publisher and author are not responsible for any health or allergy needs that may require medical supervision and are not liable for any damages or negative consequences from any treatment, action, application or preparation, to any person reading or following the information in this book.